All About Prostate Cancer

Dr. Sheila Harrison

Disclaimer

This content serves to provide general information about the disease and aims to empower you to seek prompt medical assistance if necessary to prevent complications. It's essential to stress that this information is not a substitute for consulting a qualified physician. The field of medical science is continually evolving, and due to the dynamic nature of medical knowledge, we recommend seeking expert advice if you encounter any inconsistencies or intend to take action based on the information in this content. Never disregard professional medical guidance or delay treatment based on something you've read online, including this material, or from any other online source. Always remember that the internet cannot cure you; rather, healing comes through the guidance of medical professionals and the providence of God.

Table of Content

Overview

In men and those who are assigned male at birth, prostate cancer originates in the prostate gland, which is a component of the reproductive system. Due to the fact that prostate cancer typically grows slowly and remains in the gland, many people opt for active surveillance, or no treatment. Radiation and surgery are common therapies for malignancies that develop quickly and spread. Let's take a closer look at the prostate and its functions before moving on.

The prostate is a little organ with a walnut-like form. It is in front of your rectum and beneath your bladder. Its main jobs during ejaculation are to produce fluids in your semen and push it through your urethra. It's typical for your prostate to enlarge as you get older. The second most prevalent cancer to strike men and women AMAB is prostate cancer. After 50, it's a good idea to have frequent prostate screenings. See your doctor if you experience any symptoms that point to a prostate problem.

Section 1

Prostate

A little gland that is a component of the male reproductive system is the prostate. For men and those who are assigned male at birth, the prostate gland is located in front of the rectum and underneath the bladder (AMAB). It is made up of glandular tissues and connective tissues. Its muscles aid in pushing semen through your urethra and add fluid to semen. Prostate-related conditions include benign prostatic hyperplasia, prostatitis, and malignancy.

Prostate

Cross section of the pelvis

The muscles in your prostate aid in ejaculation, and your prostate produces the fluids in your semen.

Function of Prostate

What prostate does for a men

Your ejaculate, or semen, contains extra fluid from your prostate. When you orgasm, whitish-gray fluid known as ejaculate is released from your penis. The fluid nourishes sperm cells and lubricates your urethra (pronounced "yer-ree-thruh") with enzymes, zinc, and citric acid. Your body excretes urine and ejaculate through a canal called the urethra.

When you orgasm, the muscles in your prostate also assist in pushing semen into and through your urethra.

Do females have prostate?

No, the prostate is absent in females. Skene's glands are seen in women and those who were designated female at birth (AFAB). Skene's glands, however, are sometimes referred to as the female prostate gland.

The urethra has two Skene's glands on either side of it. These glands are thought by medical experts to generate a fluid that facilitates cleaning and urination. They might serve a purpose in sexual activity as well, perhaps supplying the fluid needed for female ejaculation.

Anatomy of Prostate

The prostate's location within the body

Your prostate is located in front of your rectum and beneath your bladder. Your prostate's core is where your urethra passes.

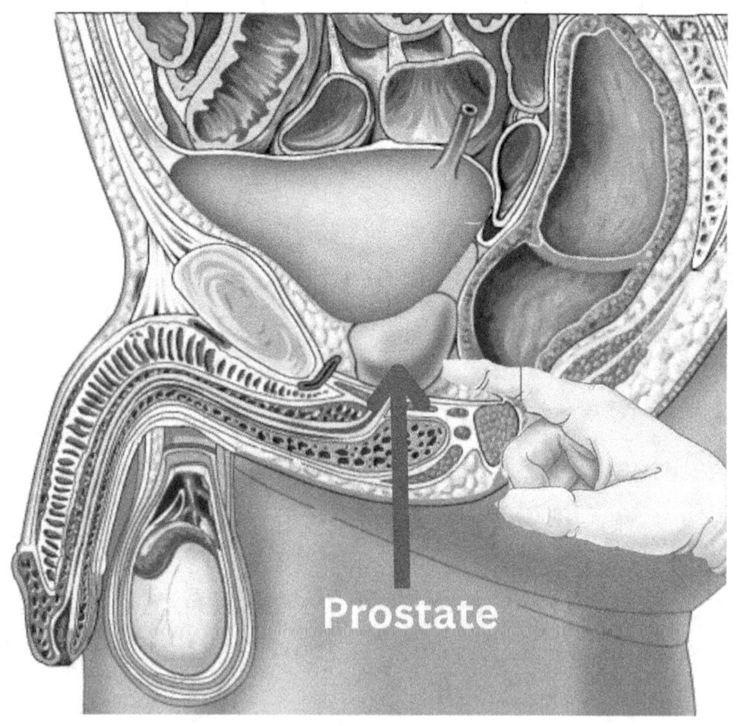

What does the prostate look like?

The prostate consists of five lobes: one median lobe located in the middle, two lateral lobes on the sides, and anterior and posterior lobes located in the front and back, respectively. It is made up of glandular tissues and connective tissues. Your prostatic fascia surrounds the prostate. The prostatic fascia is a pliable layer of connective tissue.

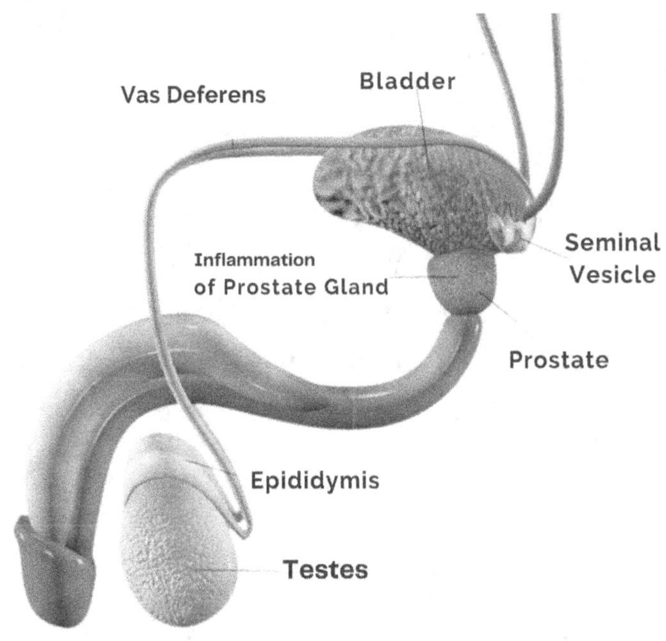

Size of Prostate

Your prostate is about the size of a walnut.

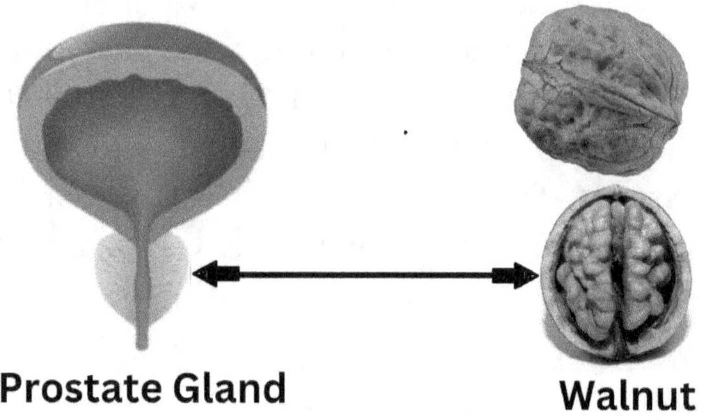

Benign prostatic hyperplasia, or the enlargement of the prostate, typically occurs after age 40. It has the ability to grow to the size of a lemon or a walnut. BPH, or benign prostatic hyperplasia, is not malignant and does not raise your chance of getting prostate cancer.

Prostate Weight

The approximate weight of your prostate is one ounce (30 grams), or five US quarters..

Conditions and Disorders

Prostate-related illnesses and ailments that are common

Common conditions that affect your prostate include:

- **Prostate cancer:** The second most prevalent disease to strike men and those who identify as male at birth is prostate cancer (AMAB).

- **Inflammation (prostatitis):** There are four types of prostatitis that can inflame your prostate gland: asymptomatic inflammatory prostatitis, chronic bacterial prostatitis, acute bacterial prostatitis, and chronic pelvic pain syndrome (CPPS). For both men and AMAB individuals under 50, it is the most prevalent urinary tract problem, while for those over 50, it ranks third.

- **Benign prostatic hyperplasia:**BPH makes your prostate enlarge, which may result in urethral obstructions. As they age, almost all males and people with AMAB will experience some prostate enlargement.

Warning Signs of Prostate Problems

Common warning signs of prostate problems include:

- Pain in your penis, testicles or perineum (pronounced "pare-uh-nee-um"). The perineum is the area between your testicles and your rectum.
- Frequent urges to pee.
- Pain while peeing (dysuria) or ejaculating.
- Slowness or dribbling of your pee stream.
- Difficulty starting to pee.
- Frequent need to get up at night to pee.
- Erectile dysfunction (ED).
- Blood in urine or semen (hematospermia).
- Pain in your lower back, hip or chest.

Common tests that check the health of the prostate

Common tests to check your prostate health include:

- **Digital rectal exam:** Your healthcare provider inserts a gloved, lubricated finger into your rectum and feels your prostate gland. Bumps or hard areas may indicate cancer.

- **Prostate-specific antigen blood test:** Your prostate makes a protein called protein-specific antigen (PSA). Elevated PSA levels may indicate cancer. PSA levels may also rise if you have BPH or prostatitis.

- **Biopsy:** Your healthcare provider uses a needle to get a sample of your prostate tissue. A healthcare provider will examine the sample under a microscope in a lab.

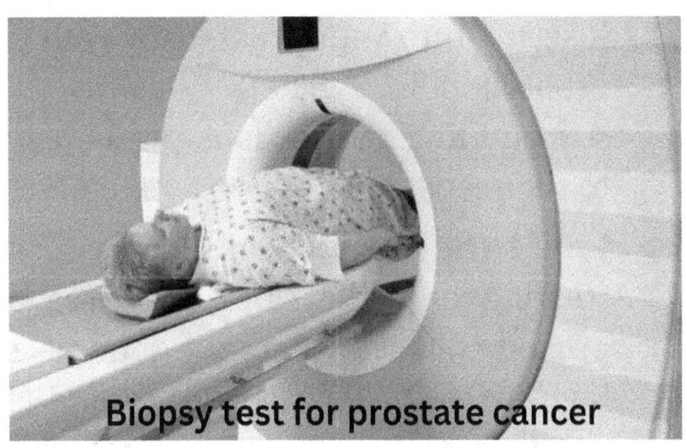

Biopsy test for prostate cancer

Treatments for Prostate

Prostate treatment depends on the type of condition you have.

Prostate cancer

- **Active surveillance:** To track the progression of cancer, you have screenings, scans, and biopsies every one to three years.

- **Brachytherapy:**Inside radiation treatment comes in the form of brachytherapy. Radiation seeds are inserted into your prostate by your medical professional. The healthy tissue surrounding the seeds is preserved thanks to the seeds.

- **Focal therapy:** Focal therapy focuses on treating only the cancerous area of your prostate. Focal therapy options include high-intensity focused ultrasound (HIFU), cryotherapy, laser ablation and photodynamic therapy (PDT).

- **Prostatectomy:** Your healthcare provider surgically removes your prostate.

Prostatitis

Your healthcare professional may suggest the following depending on the type and cause of your prostatitis:

- **Medications:** Some medications help relax the muscles around your prostate and bladder to help improve urine flow. Antibiotics help kill infection-causing bacteria.

- **Stress management:** Counseling for anxiety and depression can help relieve symptoms.

- **Exercises:** Pelvic floor exercises can help reduce or eliminate muscle spasms.

Benign prostatic hyperplasia

- **Medications:** The hormones that drive your prostate to grow can be inhibited by medication.

- **Surgery:** The prostate tissue that is preventing urine flow can be removed surgically.

- **Water vapor therapy:**An instrument is inserted into your prostate by a medical professional through your urethra. The device releases steam vapor, which reduces your prostate and destroys prostate cells.

Keeping Your prostate healthy

Help keep your prostate healthy by:

- **Prostate screenings on a regular basis:** Most persons should begin tests at age 50. Starting tests early is a good idea if there is a family history of prostate cancer..

- **Regular exercise:** Those who engage in more physical activity have a lower risk of developing BPH.

- **Eating a healthy diet:** Consuming the appropriate quantity of fruits, vegetables, and lean protein may aid in the promotion of prostate health.

- **Giving up tobacco products:** Smoking goods may raise your chance of prostate cancer.

Can I get a healthier prostate with supplements?

There isn't much information available on dietary supplements because they are exempt from FDA approval requirements and do not need to undergo clinical trials. The majority of people won't experience an improvement in their prostate health from using supplements, however they might have some tiny benefits.

Additional Common Questions

Can you live without a prostate?

It is possible to survive without a prostate.

Your doctor and you may decide to remove your prostate gland entirely if you have prostate cancer. Prostate absence is frequently accompanied by ED and involuntary urination.

How is my prostate felt?

Although you cannot touch your prostate, you can feel it either internally through your rectum or externally from the outside of your body. The rear portion of your perineum, which is closest to your rectum, is the best place to feel your prostate. Not tissue, but nerves and veins predominate in this location. You should feel a soft, rubbery prostate.

Additionally, your rectum allows you to feel your prostate more directly. About two inches of your rectum are occupied by your prostate. It feels rubbery or mushy and is located between your penis and your rectum.

The need to urinate may strike suddenly if you touch your prostate either internally or externally.

Prostate stimulation is sexually pleasurable to many people. However, a self-examination is not a reliable way to assess the health of your prostate. Speak with a medical expert if you have any worries regarding the health of your prostate. They are able to precisely evaluate the situation of your prostate and respond to any of your inquiries.

The prostate is a little organ with a walnut-like form. It is in front of your rectum and beneath your bladder. Its main jobs during ejaculation are to produce fluids in your semen and push it through your urethra. It's typical for your prostate to enlarge as you get older. The second most prevalent cancer to strike men and women AMAB is prostate cancer. After 50, it's a good idea to have frequent prostate screenings. See your doctor if you experience any symptoms that point to a prostate problem.

Section 2

Prostate Cancer

The prostate, a little walnut-shaped gland found in men and those who were assigned male at birth (AMAB), is where prostate cancer begins to grow. It is situated in front of the rectum and beneath the bladder. This little gland secretes a fluid that combines with semen to maintain the health of sperm during fertilization and pregnancy.

One dangerous condition is prostate cancer. Fortunately, the majority of prostate cancer patients receive a diagnosis prior to the cancerous cells leaving the prostate gland. This stage of treatment usually results in cancer elimination.

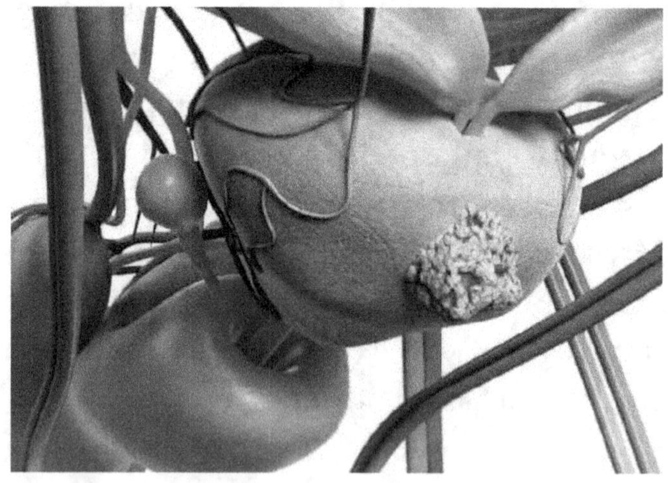

Cancerous cell developing on the Prostate gland

Types of Prostate Cancer

Adenocarcinoma is the most common type of cancer that is identified when prostate cancer is present. The glands that border your organs are where it begins. Prostate, lung, pancreatic, stomach, and colorectal cancers are among the common types of adenocarcinomas. Like your prostate, other glands that release fluid can develop adenocarcinomas in their cells. Seldom do different kinds of cells give rise to prostate cancer.

Less common types of prostate cancers include:

- Small cell carcinomas.

- Transitional cell carcinomas.

- Neuroendocrine tumors.

- Sarcomas.

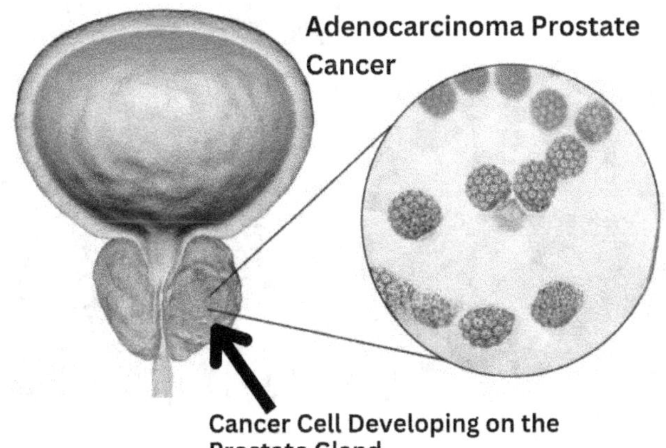

How common is prostate cancer?

The most prevalent cancer to affect men and persons AMAB is prostate cancer, which is second only to skin cancer in frequency. The U.S. Centers for Disease Control and Prevention (CDC) estimate that 13 persons out of every 100 who have prostates will eventually get prostate cancer. The majority will have regular lives and pass away from causes unrelated to prostate cancer in the end. Some people won't require care.

Nevertheless, prostate cancer claims the lives of almost 34,000 Americans every year.

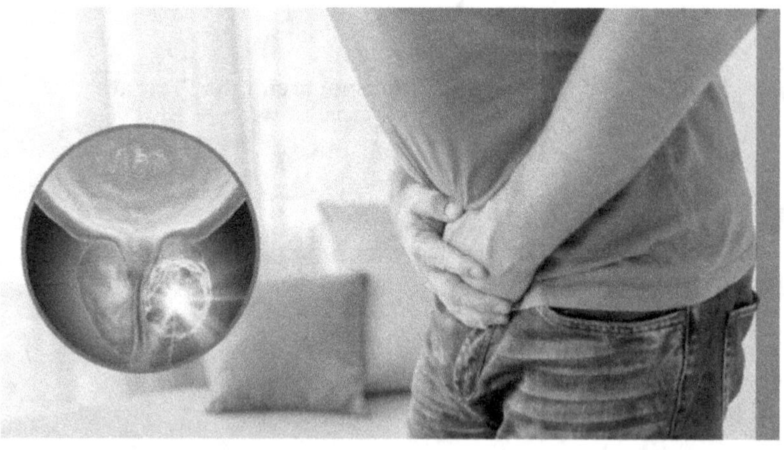

Symptoms and Causes

Symptoms of prostate cancer

The majority of prostate cancers develop gradually inside the prostate gland.

Seldom do symptoms arise from prostate cancer in its early stages. As the condition worsens, several problems could arise:

- Frequent urination, sometimes urgent, especially at night
- Weak urine flow or flow that starts and stops.
- Pain or burning when you pee (dysuria).
- Loss of bladder control (urinary incontinence).

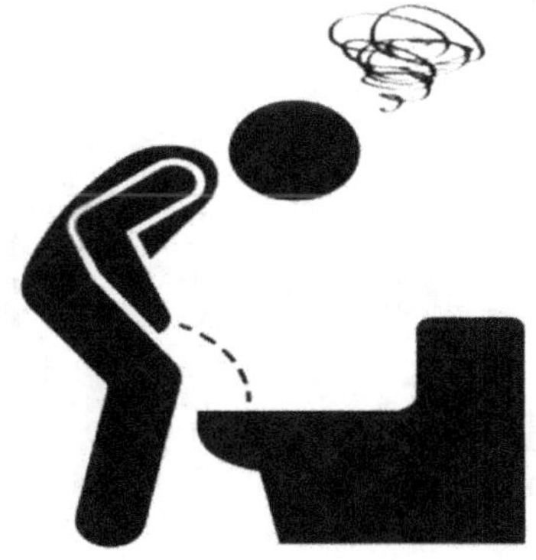

- Loss of bowel control (fecal incontinence).
- Painful ejaculation and erectile dysfunction (ED).

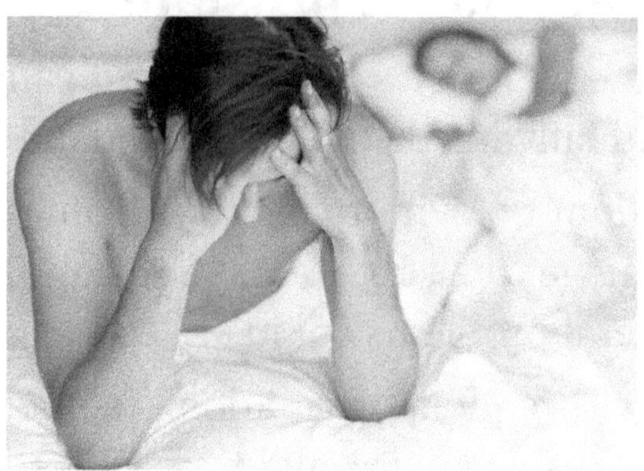

- Blood in semen (hematospermia) or pee.
- Pain in your low back, hip or chest.

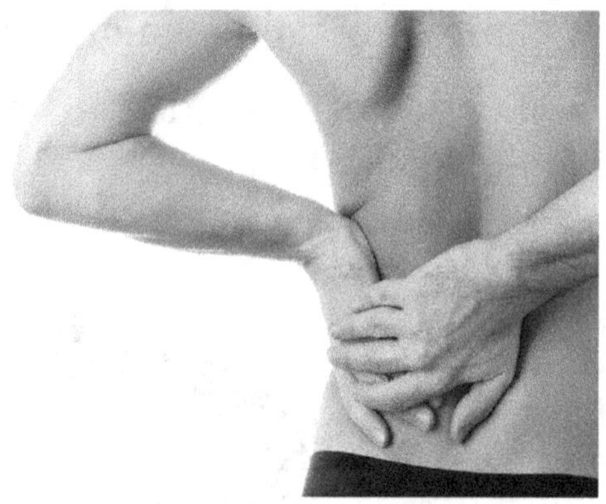

Do issues with the prostate usually indicate prostate cancer?

Not every prostatic development is cancerous. The following illnesses might also produce symptoms resembling those of prostate cancer:

- **Benign prostatic hyperplasia (BPH):** Nearly all men with prostates eventually have benign prostatic hyperplasia (BPH). Your prostate gland enlarges as a result of this disorder, but your risk of cancer does not rise.

- **Prostatitis:** An enlarged prostate gland is most likely prostatitis if you are under 50. A benign illness called prostatitis makes your prostate gland expand and inflame. Infections with bacteria are frequently the reason.

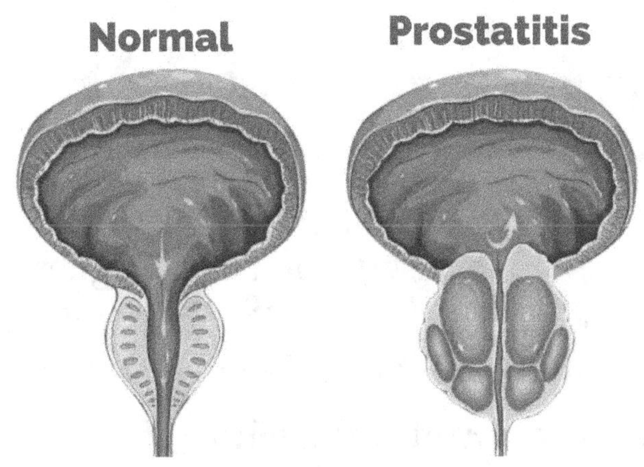

Causes Prostate Cancer

What triggers cells in your prostate to turn into cancerous ones is unknown to experts. Prostate cancer arises from abnormally fast cell division, just like other types of cancer. Cancer cells do not finally perish, in contrast to normal cells. Rather, they develop and proliferate into a bulge known as a tumor. The tumor may fragment and spread to other areas of your body as the cells become larger (metastasize).

Fortunately, prostate cancer often spreads slowly. Before the cancer has gone past your prostate, the majority of tumors are diagnosed. This stage of prostate cancer is highly curable.

Risk factors for prostate cancer

The most common risk factors include:

- **Age:** Growing older raises your risk. If you're over 50, you have a higher chance of being diagnosed. Prostate cancer affects adults over 65 in about 60% of cases.

- **Race and ethnicity:** If you're African American or Black, your chances are higher. Prostate tumors that are more prone to spread are more likely to occur in you. Prostate cancer is also more likely to develop in people under 50.

- **Family history of prostate cancer:** If a close relative already has prostate cancer, your chances of developing it are two to three times higher.

- **Genetics:** Lynch syndrome and hereditary mutations in the BRCA1 and BRCA2 genes, which are linked to an elevated risk of breast cancer, put you at higher risk.

Although the evidence is conflicting, some studies have found additional risk factors for prostate cancer. Among the other possible risk factors are:

- Smoking.

- Prostatitis.

- Having a BMI > 30 (having obesity).

- Sexually transmitted infections (STIs).

- Exposure to Agent Orange (a chemical used during the Vietnam War).

Diagnosis and Tests

Prostate Cancer diagnosis

Tests can aid in the early detection of prostate cancer. You will most likely have your first screening test at age 55 if your risk is average. If you belong to a high-risk category, you might require testing early. Typically, screenings end around age 70.

Should screenings reveal that you may have prostate cancer, you might require more testing or procedures.

Screening tests for prostate cancer

Screening tests can show whether you have signs of prostate cancer that require more testing.

- **Digital rectal exam:** Your provider inserts a gloved, lubricated finger into your rectum and feels your prostate gland. Bumps or hard areas may mean cancer.

- **Prostate-specific antigen (PSA) blood test:** The prostate gland makes a protein called protein-specific antigen (PSA).

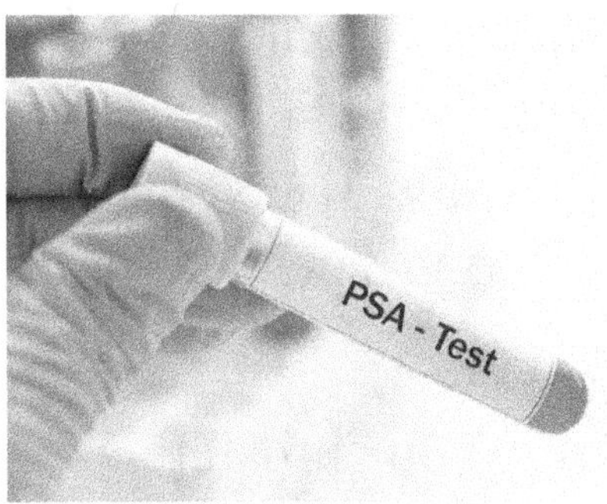

High PSA levels may indicate cancer. Levels also rise if you have benign conditions, such as BPH or prostatitis.

Diagnostic procedures for prostate cancer

A conclusive diagnosis of prostate cancer is not necessary for everyone who most likely has it. For instance, if your doctor believes that your tumor is not developing quickly enough to necessitate therapy, they can decide to postpone additional testing. If it's more aggressive—that is, developing quickly or spreading—you could require extra testing, such as a biopsy.

A conclusive diagnosis of prostate cancer is not necessary for everyone who most likely has it. For instance, your doctor might decide not to order additional tests if your tumor is judged to be slowly growing and not significant enough to need treatment. If it's more aggressive—that is, developing quickly or spreading—you could require extra testing, such as a biopsy.

- **Imaging:** Your prostate gland can be seen on an MRI or transrectal ultrasound, along with any suspicious spots that might be cancerous. Your provider may use the results of your imaging tests to determine whether to do a biopsy.

- **Biopsy:** A tissue sample is taken during a needle biopsy by a medical professional in order to test it for malignancy in a lab. The sole reliable method for determining the exact aggressiveness of prostate cancer is through a biopsy. Utilizing the biopsied tissue, your physician could run genetic tests. Certain cancer cells respond more favorably to particular treatments because of certain traits (such as mutations).

Grades and stages of prostate cancer

The Gleason score and cancer staging are used by medical professionals to assess the extent of your cancer and the kinds of therapies you require.

Gleason score

Your provider can assess the abnormality of your cancer cells using the Gleason score. Your Gleason score increases with the number of abnormal cells you have. Your provider can assess the aggressiveness or grade of your cancer by looking at the Gleason score.

Staging prostate cancer

Your healthcare professional can assess the extent of your cancer's spread and how far along it is by doing cancer staging. You may have localized cancer in your prostate gland, regional cancer that invades surrounding structures, or metastatic cancer that spreads to other organs. The lymph nodes and bones are the most typical places where prostate cancer spreads. Along with other organs, your liver, brain, and lungs may also develop it.

Management and Treatment

Treatment and Management of Prostate Cancer

Your overall health, the presence and rate of cancerous growth, and other factors will all affect your course of therapy. Urologists, radiation oncologists, and medical oncologists are just a few of the healthcare professionals you might collaborate with, depending on your course of treatment. Treatment is available for most cases of early-stage prostate cancer diagnosis.

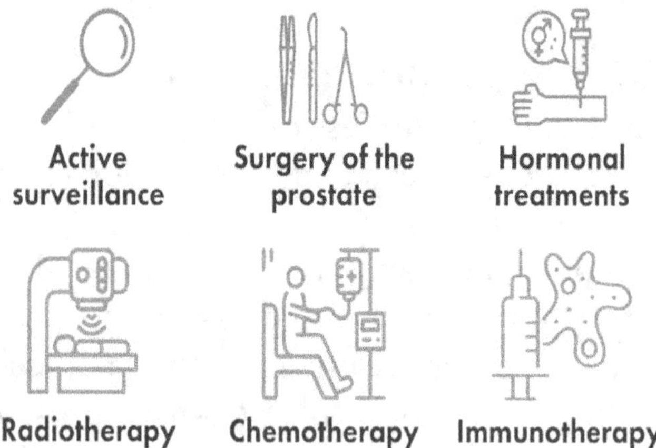

Specific procedures used

Surveillance

If your cancer grows slowly and doesn't spread, your doctor can choose to watch you rather than treat you.

- **Active surveillance:** Every one to three years, you undergo screenings, scans, and biopsies to track the progression of cancer. If the cancer is limited to your prostate, grows slowly, and is not causing symptoms, active surveillance is most effective. Your physician may begin treatment if your problem gets worse.

- **Watchful waiting:** While watchful waiting and active surveillance are comparable, watchful waiting is more frequently employed for cancer patients who are fragile and unlikely to improve with treatment. Testing occurs far less frequently as well. Treatments typically concentrate on symptom management rather than tumor elimination.

Surgery

A damaged prostate gland is removed during a radical prostatectomy. When a prostate cancer is effectively removed, it usually does not spread. If your surgeon thinks you would benefit from this procedure, they can advise you on the optimal removal technique.

- **Open radical prostatectomy:** Your prostate gland is removed by your physician through a single abdominal incision that runs from your belly button to your pubic bone. Compared to less invasive procedures like robotic prostatectomy, this technique is less common.

- **Robotic radical prostatectomy:** Using a robotic radical prostatectomy, your surgeon can operate through multiple microscopic incisions. They use a console to control a robot system rather than working directly.

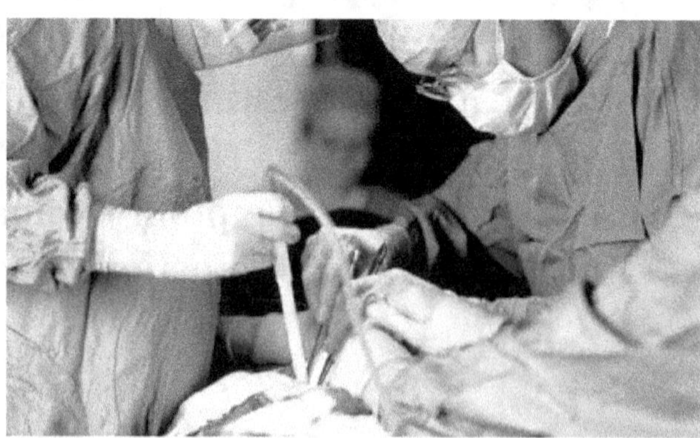

Radiation Therapy

Radiation therapy may be used alone or in conjunction with other treatments to treat prostate cancer. Additionally, radiation can relieve symptoms.

- **Brachytherapy:** Brachytherapy is a type of internal radiation therapy in which radioactive seeds are inserted into your prostate. With this method, cancer cells are eliminated without harming the surrounding healthy tissue.

- **External beam radiation therapy:** Strong X-ray beams are directed toward the tumor by a machine during external beam radiation therapy (EBRT). High radiation doses can be directed at the tumor with specialized EBRT techniques like IMRT, all while protecting healthy tissue.

Systemic therapies

If the cancer has progressed outside of your prostate gland, your physician might suggest systemic treatments. With systemic therapy, chemicals are delivered throughout your body to either kill or stop the growth of cancer cells.

- **Hormone therapy:** Testosterone stimulates the proliferation of cancer cells. Medication is used in hormone therapy to counteract testosterone's effect in promoting the growth of cancer cells. The medications function by either lowering your testosterone levels or blocking testosterone from reaching cancer cells. As an alternative, your doctor can advise an orchiectomy, which involves removing your testicles to stop them from producing testosterone. Those who would prefer not to take medication can choose to get this operation.

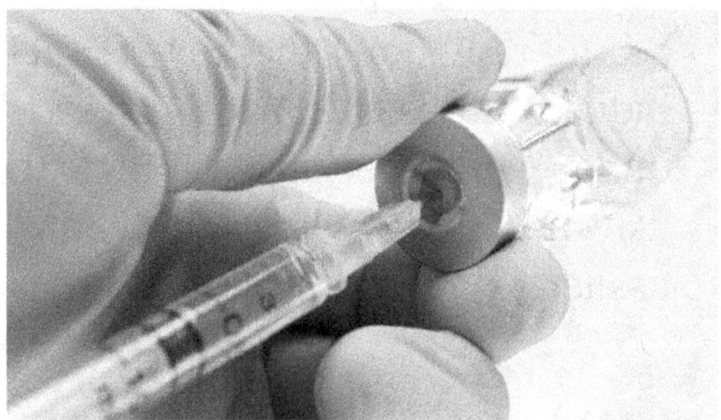

- **Chemotherapy:** Chemotherapy kills cancer cells with medication. If your cancer has progressed beyond your prostate, you may be treated with hormone therapy in addition to chemotherapy.

- **Immunotherapy:** Your immune system becomes stronger with immunotherapy, making it more capable of recognizing and combating cancer cells. Immunotherapy may be suggested by your doctor to treat advanced cancer or recurrent cancer, which is cancer that disappears for a while before coming back.

- **Targeted therapy:** In order to stop cancerous cells from proliferating, targeted therapy focuses on the genetic alterations (mutations) that cause healthy cells to become cancerous cells. Prostate cancer patients who have BRCA gene mutations are treated with targeted treatments that kill cancer cells.

Focal therapy

A more recent type of treatment that eliminates malignancies inside your prostate is called focal therapy. This treatment may be suggested by your healthcare practitioner in the event that the cancer is low-risk and has not spread. Many of these medical procedures are still regarded as experimental.

- **High-intensity focused ultrasound (HIFU):** Strong heat produced by high-intensity sound waves destroys prostate cancer cells.

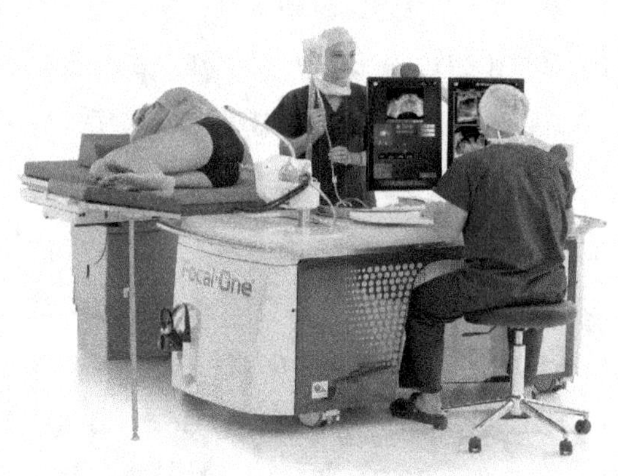

- **Cryotherapy:** Your prostate's cancer cells are frozen by cold gasses, which removes the tumor.

- **Laser ablation:** Intense heat directed at the tumor kills cancer cells within your prostate, destroying the tumor.

- **Photodynamic therapy:** Medications make cancer cells more sensitive to certain wavelengths of light. A healthcare provider exposes cancer cells to these light wavelengths, killing the cancer cells.

Side effects of prostate cancer treatment

Potential side effects include:

- **Incontinence:** When you laugh, cough, or feel the sudden urge to urinate even when your bladder isn't full, you can leak pee. Without treatment, this issue often gets better throughout the first six to twelve months.

- **Erectile dysfunction (ED):** The erectile nerves in your penis can be damaged by radiation, surgery, and other medical procedures, which can impair your ability to achieve and sustain an erection. Regaining erectile function usually takes a year or two, sometimes even less time. Medication like tadalafil (Cialis®) or sildenafil (Viagra®) can help in the interim by boosting blood flow to your penis.

- **Infertility:** Infertility might arise from treatments that interfere with your capacity to ejaculate or make sperm. Before beginning therapy, you can store sperm in a sperm bank if you want children in the future. Sperm extraction may be necessary after treatments. Sperm from testicular tissue are extracted specifically for this surgery and then placed into your partner's uterus.

If you're having side affects from your medication, speak with your doctor. They can frequently suggest treatments and medications that can be beneficial.

Prevention

Prevention of Prostate Cancer

Prostate cancer cannot be prevented. However, following these guidelines could lower your risk:

- **Get regular prostate screenings**: Based on your risk factors, find out from your healthcare practitioner how frequently you should get examined.

- **Keep a healthy weight**: Find out from your doctor what constitutes a healthy weight for you.

- **Engage in regular exercise:** The CDC suggests 150 minutes a week, or little over 20 minutes a day, of moderate-intensity activity.

- **Consume a healthy diet:** While there isn't a single diet that may prevent cancer, healthy eating practices can help you stay healthier overall. Consume entire grains, fruits, and veggies. Steer clear of processed foods and red meat.

- **Give up smoking:** Steer clear of tobacco goods. If you smoke, work through a smoking cessation program with your healthcare professional to break the habit.

Prognosis and prospects

What is the outlook (prognosis) for those suffering from prostate cancer?

If your healthcare professional finds prostate cancer early, you have a very good prognosis. Ninety-nine percent of people with prostate cancer who receive a diagnosis survive for at least five years following their diagnosis.

When prostate cancer has metastasized, or spread outside of the prostate, survival odds are lower. After five years, 32% of patients with metastatic prostate cancer are still alive.

How treatable is prostate cancer?

Yes, if it's discovered quickly. Sometimes cancer progresses so slowly that treatment may not be necessary immediately away. Prostate cancers that have not progressed outside of the prostate gland can frequently be cured with treatment.

When to see your Doctor

You should call your healthcare provider if you experience:

- Difficulty peeing.
- Peeing frequently (incontinence).
- Pain when you pee or have intercourse.
- Blood in your pee or semen.

Questions you should ask Your Doctor

If you have prostate cancer, you may want to ask your healthcare provider:

- Has the cancer spread outside of my prostate gland?
- What's the best treatment for the stage of prostate cancer I have?
- What are the treatment risks and side effects?
- Is my family at risk for developing prostate cancer? If so, should we get genetic tests?
- What kind of follow-up care do I need after treatment?

- Should I look out for signs of complications?

Prostate cancer is often very treatable with early diagnosis and care. Many patients who receive a diagnosis while the cancer hasn't progressed past their prostate go on to lead healthy, cancer-free lives for a number of years after therapy. However, a tiny percentage of individuals may experience an aggressive sickness that spreads swiftly to other body areas. Based on your risk factors, your healthcare professional can advise you on the optimal screening regimen. They can advise on the most effective course of action depending on how aggressively or slowly your cancer is developing.